INSULIN RESISTANCE COOKBOOK FOR SENIORS

Quick and easy recipes to lose weight, manage insulin sensitivity and prevent prediabetes

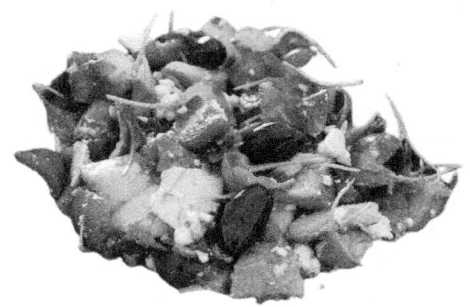

Dr. Malvin Harison

Copyright © by Dr. Malvin Harison 2023. All rights reserved.

Before this document is duplicated or reproduced in any manner, the publisher's consent must be gained. Therefore, the contents within can neither be stored electronically, transferred, nor kept in a database. Neither in Part nor full can the document be copied, scanned, faxed, or retained without approval from the publisher or creator.

TABLE OF CONTENT

Introduction   4
   Overview   6
   Preventive Measures   7

Chapter 1: The Importance of Diet in Managing Insulin Resistance   8
   Understanding Insulin Resistance and its Dietary Connection   9
   Carbohydrates and Glycemic Index   9
   Balancing Macronutrients   10
   Nutrient-Dense Foods   11
   Fruits and Vegetables Recommendations   11
   Omega-3 Fatty Acids   12
   The Impact of Lifestyle and Dietary Habits on Insulin Resistance   12
   Crafting a Senior-Focused Insulin Resistance Diet   14
   Adapting Recipes for Seniors   14
   Mindful Eating for Seniors   15
   Complications of the disease if diet is not taken 16
   Foods to Eat with benefits   18
   Foods to Limit or Avoid with reasons   20

Chapter 2: Healthy and delicious breakfast Recipes   23
   1. Quinoa Breakfast Bowl   23
   2. Greek Yogurt Parfait   24
   3. Avocado and Egg Toast   25
   4. Chia Seed Pudding   26
   5. Spinach and Feta Omelette   27

6. Sweet Potato Hash with Turkey Sausage	29
7. Berry and Almond Smoothie Bowl	30
8. Cottage Cheese and Pineapple Parfait	31
9. Mushroom and Spinach Breakfast Wrap	32
10. Peanut Butter Banana Overnight Oats	33
Chapter 3: Satisfying Lunch Recipes	**34**
1. Grilled Salmon Salad	34
2. Quinoa and Vegetable Stir-Fry	35
3. Chicken and Vegetable Wrap	36
4. Sweet Potato and Chickpea Buddha Bowl	37
5. Mediterranean Hummus Plate	38
6. Turkey and Quinoa Stuffed Bell Peppers	39
7. Salmon and Avocado Wrap	40
8. Caprese Salad with Balsamic Glaze	41
9. Shrimp and Quinoa Salad	43
10. Vegetarian Lentil Soup	44
Chapter 4: Colorful Dinner	**45**
1. Grilled Chicken and Vegetable Skewers	45
2. Vegetarian Stuffed Bell Peppers	46
3. Salmon and Asparagus Foil Packets	47
4. Eggplant and Chickpea Curry	49
5. Turkey and Vegetable Stir-Fry	50
6. Cauliflower and Chickpea Curry	51
7. Shrimp and Zucchini Noodles	52
8. Chickpea and Spinach Stew	53
9. Teriyaki Tofu Stir-Fry	55
10. Mushroom and Lentil Stuffed Peppers	56
Chapter 4: Nutrient-rich Snacks	**57**
1. Greek Yogurt and Berry Parfait	57
2. Apple Slices with Almond Butter	58

3. Vegetable Sticks with Hummus	60
4. Hard-Boiled Eggs with Avocado	61
5. Trail Mix	61
6. Cottage Cheese with Pineapple	62
7. Rice Cake with Almond Butter and Banana Slices	63
8. Yogurt-Dipped Strawberries	64
9. Edamame Pods	64
10. Dark Chocolate and Almond Clusters	65
Chapter 6:Bonus 1: 7-day meal plan	**67**
Day 1	67
Day 2	67
Day 3	67
Day 4	68
Day 5	68
Day 6	69
Day 7	69
Chapter 7: Bonus 2: Insulin resistance Juicing and Smoothie Recipes for seniors	**71**
1. Green Detox Juice	71
2. Beetroot Blast	71
3. Citrus Burst Juice	71
4. Carrot-Orange Elixir	72
5. Cucumber Mint Cooler	72
6. Berry Bliss Smoothie	72
7. Pineapple Paradise	73
8. Green Power Smoothie	73
9. Avocado Delight	73
10. Mango Tango Smoothie	74
11. Berries and Oats Smoothie	74

12. Chia-Berry Protein Smoothie	74
13. Spinach and Banana Smoothie	75
14. Kiwi-Citrus Crush	75
15. Strawberry Almond Bliss	75
16. Turmeric Golden Smoothie	76
17. Peachy Green Smoothie	76
18. Blueberry Lavender Refresher	76
19. Apple Pie Smoothie	77
20. Pomegranate Berry Blast	77
Conclusion	77

Introduction

Welcome to the "Insulin Resistance Diet Cookbook for Seniors," a comprehensive guide designed to empower seniors in managing and preventing insulin resistance through a wholesome and enjoyable approach to nutrition.

In the golden years of life, prioritizing health becomes paramount, and this cookbook aims to be your trusted companion on the journey to optimal well-being.

Overview

As we age, our bodies undergo various changes, and one significant concern for seniors is insulin resistance. Insulin resistance occurs when the body's cells become less responsive to insulin, a hormone responsible for regulating blood sugar levels. This condition can lead to an increased risk of type 2 diabetes, cardiovascular issues, and other health complications.

This cookbook is tailored to address the unique dietary needs of seniors dealing with insulin resistance. By incorporating nutrient-dense and balanced recipes, we aim to promote stable blood sugar levels, enhance energy levels, and support overall health. Each recipe has been carefully crafted to provide not only delicious meals but also to aid in managing insulin resistance effectively.

Preventive Measures

Prevention is often the best medicine. This cookbook not only serves as a collection of delectable recipes but also as a guide to adopting preventive measures against insulin resistance. We explore lifestyle choices, exercise routines, and habits that can significantly reduce the risk of insulin resistance and its associated complications.

The Preventive Measures section provides practical advice on maintaining a healthy lifestyle, including exercise regimens suitable for seniors, stress management techniques, and tips for adequate sleep. By adopting these measures, you can proactively enhance your well-being and decrease the likelihood of developing insulin resistance.

Chapter 1: The Importance of Diet in Managing Insulin Resistance

In the intricate tapestry of health and well-being, diet stands out as a cornerstone, particularly when it comes to managing insulin resistance. Insulin resistance, a condition where cells become less responsive to insulin's regulatory signals, is intricately linked to diet and nutrition.

This comprehensive exploration delves into the vital role that diet plays in the development, management, and prevention of insulin resistance, especially in the context of seniors.

Understanding Insulin Resistance and its Dietary Connection

Insulin, a hormone produced by the pancreas of the liver, plays a very vital role in regulating the level of blood sugar in the body. When cells develop resistance to insulin, the body struggles to efficiently utilize glucose, leading to elevated blood sugar levels. The foods we consume directly impact this intricate dance between insulin and glucose.

Carbohydrates and Glycemic Index

One of the key dietary considerations in managing insulin resistance is the type and quality of carbohydrates consumed. Foods with a high glycemic index can cause rapid spikes in blood sugar levels, putting increased demand on insulin. This emphasizes the importance of choosing complex carbohydrates, such as whole grains, legumes, and vegetables, which are digested more slowly and help maintain stable blood sugar levels.

Balancing Macronutrients

The balance between macronutrients—carbohydrates, proteins, and fats—is crucial for individuals with insulin resistance. A well-balanced diet helps regulate blood sugar levels and promotes satiety. Incorporating lean proteins, healthy fats, and complex carbohydrates in appropriate proportions can contribute to better blood sugar control.

Nutrient-Dense Foods

The concept of nutrient density is paramount in crafting a diet that supports insulin sensitivity. Nutrient-dense foods provide essential vitamins, minerals, and antioxidants without excess calories or refined sugars.

Seniors, in particular, benefit from a diet rich in nutrient-dense options to meet their unique nutritional needs.

Fruits and Vegetables Recommendations

Colorful fruits and vegetables are packed with antioxidants and fiber, offering a myriad of health benefits. These foods not only support overall well-being but also contribute to improved insulin sensitivity. Berries, leafy greens, and cruciferous vegetables are especially noteworthy additions to an insulin-friendly diet.

Omega-3 Fatty Acids

Incorporating sources of omega-3 fatty acids, such as fatty fish, flaxseeds, and walnuts, can be advantageous in managing insulin resistance. These essential fats possess anti-inflammatory properties and may contribute to improved insulin sensitivity.

The Impact of Lifestyle and Dietary Habits on Insulin Resistance

Beyond individual food choices, lifestyle and dietary habits play a pivotal role in the development and management of insulin resistance. Seniors, with their unique health considerations, can significantly benefit from adopting a holistic approach to their well-being.

Physical Activity: Regular physical activity is a cornerstone of insulin sensitivity. Exercise helps muscles utilize glucose more efficiently, reducing the burden on insulin. Tailored exercise regimens for seniors, including aerobic activities, resistance training, and flexibility exercises, can contribute to better blood sugar control and overall health.

Meal Timing and Frequency: The timing and frequency of meals also influence insulin sensitivity.

Eating smaller, balanced meals throughout the day can help regulate blood sugar levels, preventing dramatic spikes. Additionally, incorporating mindful eating practices, such as savoring each bite and paying attention to hunger and fullness cues, can positively impact insulin response.

Crafting a Senior-Focused Insulin Resistance Diet

Recognizing the distinct needs of seniors, a tailored approach to diet becomes imperative. The "Insulin Resistance Diet Cookbook for Seniors" serves as a valuable resource, offering a diverse array of recipes that not only cater to nutritional requirements but also delight the taste buds.

Adapting Recipes for Seniors

The cookbook emphasizes the incorporation of nutrient-dense, senior-friendly ingredients. From easy-to-prepare breakfast options to satisfying main courses and delightful desserts, each recipe is crafted to provide essential nutrients while considering factors such as digestion, taste preferences, and overall health.

Mindful Eating for Seniors

The cookbook also encourages a mindful approach to eating. By savoring flavors, appreciating textures, and enjoying meals in a relaxed setting, seniors can enhance the overall dining experience and potentially improve digestion and nutrient absorption.

Complications of the disease if diet is not taken

Failure to address insulin resistance through a balanced diet can lead to severe complications, including:

1. Type 2 Diabetes: Uncontrolled insulin resistance often progresses to type 2 diabetes, necessitating ongoing medical management.

2. Cardiovascular Issues: Elevated blood sugar levels contribute to cardiovascular problems, increasing the risk of heart disease, stroke, and hypertension.

3. Weight Gain: Insulin resistance is linked to weight gain, particularly around the abdomen, exacerbating the condition and associated health risks.

4. Chronic Inflammation: Persistent insulin resistance can trigger chronic inflammation, fostering conditions like arthritis and other inflammatory disorders.

5. Metabolic Syndrome: Insulin resistance is a key component of metabolic syndrome, a cluster of conditions heightening the risk of heart disease, stroke, and diabetes.

6. Kidney Damage: Prolonged insulin resistance may lead to kidney damage, impacting their ability to filter blood effectively.

7. Neurological Issues: Insulin resistance is implicated in cognitive decline and an increased risk of neurodegenerative disorders such as Alzheimer's disease.

8. Reproductive Complications: Women with insulin resistance may experience fertility issues, and it can contribute to complications during pregnancy.

Foods to Eat with benefits

1. Fiber-Rich Foods: Whole grains (quinoa, brown rice), legumes (beans, lentils), and fibrous vegetables (broccoli, spinach).
- **Benefits**: Fiber aids in blood sugar regulation and promotes satiety.

2. Lean Proteins: Skinless poultry, fish, tofu, eggs, and low-fat dairy.
- **Benefits**: Protein helps stabilize blood sugar levels and supports muscle health.

3. Healthy Fats: Avocado, nuts, seeds, and olive oil.

- Benefits: Monounsaturated fats contribute to heart health and help manage insulin resistance.

4. Colorful Vegetables: Bell peppers, carrots, kale, and tomatoes.
- **Benefits**: Rich in antioxidants and vitamins, supporting overall health.

5. Berries: Blueberries, strawberries, raspberries.
- Benefits: Low in sugar, high in antioxidants, and contribute to better blood sugar control.

6. Fatty Fish: Salmon, mackerel, sardines.
- Benefits: Omega-3 fatty acids support heart health and reduce inflammation.

7. Low-Glycemic Fruits: Apples, pears, cherries.

- **Benefits**: Provide sweetness with a slower impact on blood sugar.

8. Herbs and Spices: Cinnamon, turmeric, ginger.
- Benefits: Anti-inflammatory properties may aid in insulin sensitivity.

Foods to Limit or Avoid with reasons

1. Refined Carbohydrate: White bread, sugary cereals, and pastries.
- Reason: Rapidly raise blood sugar levels.

2. Processed Foods: Packaged snacks, fast food, and sugary beverages.
Reason: High in added sugars and unhealthy fats.

3. Sugary Treats: Candy, cakes, and sugary desserts.
- Reason: Contribute to blood sugar spikes.

4. Trans Fats: Margarine, partially hydrogenated oils.
- Reason: Linked to insulin resistance and heart disease.

5. High-Sodium Foods: Processed meats, canned soups.
- Reason: Excessive sodium intake may contribute to hypertension.

6. Sweetened Beverages: Soda, fruit juices with added sugars.
- Reason: Can lead to rapid increases in blood sugar.

7. Excessive Alcohol: Moderation is key.
- Reason: Alcohol can affect blood sugar levels, and excessive consumption may contribute to insulin resistance.

8. Highly Processed Meats: Bacon, sausage, and deli meats.
- Reason: Processed meats often contain additives that may impact health negatively.

Chapter 2: Healthy and delicious breakfast Recipes

Number of servings, cooking time and nutritional values inclusive

1. Quinoa Breakfast Bowl

Serving: 1 bowl
Nutritional Value
- High-quality protein from quinoa
- Fiber from quinoa and fresh berries
- Healthy fats from almonds

Cooking Time: 15 minutes
Ingredients
- 1/2 cup cooked quinoa
- 1/4 cup sliced almonds
- 1/2 cup fresh berries (blueberries, strawberries)
- 1 tablespoon honey
- 1/2 cup almond milk

Instructions

1. Combine cooked quinoa, sliced almonds, and fresh berries in a bowl.
2. Drizzle with honey and pour almond milk over the mixture.
3. Gently stir and enjoy a protein-packed, nutrient-rich breakfast.

2. Greek Yogurt Parfait

Serving: 1 parfait
Nutritional Value
- Protein from Greek yogurt
- Fiber from granola and berries
- Probiotics for gut health

Cooking Time: 10 minutes
Ingredients
- 1/2 cup Greek yogurt
- 1/4 cup granola (low sugar)
- 1/2 cup mixed berries (raspberries, blackberries)
- 1 tablespoon chia seeds

Instructions

1. In a glass, layer Greek yogurt, granola, and mixed berries.
2. Repeat the layers, finishing with a sprinkle of chia seeds.
3. Allow it to set for a few minutes before enjoying a delightful and filling parfait.

3. Avocado and Egg Toast

Serving: 1 toast
Nutritional Value
- Healthy fats from avocado
- Protein from eggs
- Fiber from whole grain toast

Cooking Time: 10 minutes
Ingredients
- 1 slice whole grain bread
- 1/2 ripe avocado, mashed
- 1 poached or fried egg
- Salt and pepper to taste

Instructions
1. Toast the whole grain bread to your liking.
2. Spread mashed avocado on the toast.

3. Top with a poached or fried egg, and season with salt and pepper.

4. Chia Seed Pudding

Serving: 1 bowl

Nutritional Value
- Omega-3 fatty acids from chia seeds
- Protein from Greek yogurt
- Fiber for digestive health

Prep Time: 5 minutes (+ overnight chilling)

Ingredients
- 2 tablespoons chia seeds
- 1/2 cup almond milk
- 1/4 cup Greek yogurt
- 1/2 teaspoon vanilla extract
- Fresh berries for topping

Instructions

1. Mix chia seeds, almond milk, Greek yogurt, and vanilla extract in a bowl.
2. Refrigerate overnight or for at least 4 hours.
3. Top with fresh berries before serving.

5. Spinach and Feta Omelette

Serving: 1 omelet

Nutritional Value
- Protein from eggs
- Iron and vitamins from spinach
- Healthy fats from feta cheese

Cooking Time: 15 minutes

Ingredients
- 2 eggs, beaten
- Handful of fresh spinach
- 2 tablespoons crumbled feta cheese
- Salt and pepper to taste

Instructions

1. In a pan, sauté spinach until wilted.
2. Pour beaten eggs over the spinach, sprinkle with feta, and season.
3. Cook until the eggs are set, then fold in half and serve.

6. Sweet Potato Hash with Turkey Sausage

Serving: 1 plate

Nutritional Value
- Fiber and vitamins from sweet potatoes
- Lean protein from turkey sausage
- Healthy fats from olive oil

Cooking Time: 20 minutes

Ingredients
- 1 small sweet potato, grated
- 2 turkey sausage links, sliced
- 1/4 cup diced bell peppers
- 1 tablespoon olive oil

Instructions

1. In a pan, heat olive oil and sauté sweet potatoes until golden.
2. Add turkey sausage and bell peppers, cooking until everything is cooked through.
3. Season to taste and serve hot.

7. Berry and Almond Smoothie Bowl

Serving: 1 bowl

Nutritional Value
- Antioxidants from berries
- Protein from almond butter
- Fiber from spinach and chia seeds

Prep Time: 10 minutes

Ingredients

- 1 cup mixed berries (strawberries, blueberries)
- 1/2 banana
- Handful of spinach
- 1 tablespoon almond butter
- 1 tablespoon chia seeds
- 1/2 cup almond milk

Instructions

1. Blend berries, banana, spinach, almond butter, chia seeds, and almond milk until smooth.
2. Pour into a bowl and top with additional berries or granola.

8. Cottage Cheese and Pineapple Parfait

Serving: 1 parfait
Nutritional Value
- Protein from cottage cheese
- Digestive enzymes from pineapple
- Fiber from granola

Prep Time: 10 minutes
Ingredients
- 1/2 cup low-fat cottage cheese
- 1/2 cup fresh pineapple chunks
- 2 tablespoons granola (low sugar)
- Drizzle of honey

Instructions
1. Layer cottage cheese, pineapple chunks, and granola in a glass.
2. Drizzle with honey and enjoy this tropical-inspired parfait.

9. Mushroom and Spinach Breakfast Wrap

Serving: 1 wrap
Nutritional Value
- Protein from eggs
- Iron and vitamins from spinach
- Fiber from whole grain wrap

Cooking Time: 15 minutes
Ingredients
- 2 eggs, scrambled
- Handful of fresh spinach
- 1/2 cup sliced mushrooms
- Whole grain wrap

Instructions
1. Sauté mushrooms until browned, add spinach until wilted, and set aside.
2. Scramble eggs and mix with the sautéed vegetables.
3. Fill a whole grain wrap with the egg and vegetable mixture, then roll up and serve.

10. Peanut Butter Banana Overnight Oats

Serving: 1 jar
Nutritional Value
- Protein from Greek yogurt and peanut butter
- Potassium and fiber from bananas
- Satiety from oats

Prep Time: 5 minutes (+ overnight chilling)

Ingredients
- 1/2 cup rolled oats
- 1/2 cup Greek yogurt
- 1/2 cup almond milk
- 1 tablespoon peanut butter
- 1/2 banana, sliced

Instructions
1. In a jar, combine rolled oats, Greek yogurt, almond milk, and peanut butter.
2. Mix well, add banana slices, and refrigerate overnight.
3. Stir before serving for a delicious, no-cook breakfast.

Chapter 3: Satisfying Lunch Recipes

1. Grilled Salmon Salad

Serving: 1 salad

Nutritional Value
- Omega-3 fatty acids from salmon
- Fiber and vitamins from leafy greens
- Healthy fats from olive oil

Cooking Time: 20 minutes

Ingredients

- 4 oz grilled salmon filet
- Mixed greens (spinach, arugula)
- Cherry tomatoes, halved
- Cucumber slices
- 1 tablespoon olive oil and balsamic vinegar dressing

Instructions

1. Grill salmon until cooked.
2. Assemble a salad with mixed greens, cherry tomatoes, cucumber slices, and grilled salmon.

3. Saute with balsamic vinegar dressing and olive oil.

2. Quinoa and Vegetable Stir-Fry

Serving: 1 bowl
Nutritional Value
- Protein from quinoa and tofu
- Fiber and vitamins from vegetables
- Healthy fats from sesame oil

Cooking Time: 25 minutes
Ingredients
- 1/2 cup cooked quinoa
- 4 oz tofu, cubed
- Broccoli florets, bell peppers, and snap peas
- 1 tablespoon sesame oil
- Low-sodium soy sauce to taste

Instructions
1. Stir-fry tofu and vegetables in sesame oil until tender.
2. Add cooked quinoa and soy sauce, mixing well.
3. Serve this nutrient-packed stir-fry bowl.

3. Chicken and Vegetable Wrap

Serving: 1 wrap

Nutritional Value
- Lean protein from chicken
- Fiber and vitamins from whole grain wrap and veggies
- Healthy fats from avocado

Cooking Time: 15 minutes

Ingredients
- Grilled chicken slices
- Whole grain wrap
- Mixed greens, tomatoes, and cucumbers
- 1/4 avocado, sliced

Instructions
1. Fill a whole grain wrap with grilled chicken, mixed greens, tomatoes, cucumbers, and avocado slices.
2. Roll up and enjoy a satisfying and nutritious wrap.

4. Sweet Potato and Chickpea Buddha Bowl

Serving: 1 bowl

Nutritional Value
- Fiber and vitamins from sweet potatoes and chickpeas
- Protein from quinoa
- Healthy fats from tahini dressing

Cooking Time: 30 minutes

Ingredients
- Roasted sweet potato cubes
- Cooked quinoa
- Chickpeas (canned, drained, and rinsed)
- Chopped kale or spinach
- Tahini dressing

Instructions
1. Assemble a bowl with roasted sweet potatoes, quinoa, chickpeas, and greens.
2. Drizzle with tahini dressing for a flavorful and nutrient-rich lunch.

5. Mediterranean Hummus Plate

Serving: 1 plate
- **Nutritional Value**

Plant-based protein from hummus
- Healthy fats from olives and olive oil
- Fiber and vitamins from vegetables

Prep Time: 15 minutes

Ingredients
- Hummus
- Cherry tomatoes, cucumber slices, and bell pepper strips
- Kalamata olives
- Feta cheese
- Drizzle of extra virgin olive oil

Instructions

1. Arrange hummus, cherry tomatoes, cucumber slices, bell pepper strips, and olives on a plate.
2. Crumble feta over the top and drizzle with extra virgin olive oil.

6. Turkey and Quinoa Stuffed Bell Peppers

Serving: 1 pepper

Nutritional Value
- Lean protein from turkey
- Fiber and vitamins from quinoa and vegetables
- Antioxidants from bell peppers

Cooking Time: 40 minutes

Ingredients

- Bell peppers, halved and cleaned
- Ground turkey
- Cooked quinoa
- Diced tomatoes and black beans
- Taco seasoning

Instructions

1. Brown turkey in a pan, add cooked quinoa, diced tomatoes, black beans, and taco seasoning.
2. Stuff bell peppers with the turkey and quinoa mixture.
3. Bake until peppers are tender and serve.

7. Salmon and Avocado Wrap

Serving: 1 wrap

Nutritional Value
- Omega-3 fatty acids from salmon
- Healthy fats from avocado
- Fiber and vitamins from whole grain wrap and veggies

Cooking Time: 15 minutes

Ingredients
- Grilled salmon
- Whole grain wrap
- Avocado slices
- Lettuce, tomato, and red onion
- Greek yogurt or tzatziki sauce

Instructions

1. Assemble a wrap with grilled salmon, avocado slices, lettuce, tomato, red onion, and a dollop of Greek yogurt or tzatziki.
2. Roll up and enjoy this flavorful and nutritious lunch.

8. Caprese Salad with Balsamic Glaze

Serving: 1 salad

Nutritional Value
- Protein from mozzarella
- Antioxidants from tomatoes and basil
- Healthy fats from olive oil

Prep Time: 10 minutes

Ingredients
- Fresh mozzarella, sliced
- Tomatoes, sliced
- Fresh basil leaves
- Drizzle of balsamic glaze
- Olive oil, salt, and pepper to taste

Instructions

1. Arrange mozzarella slices, tomato slices, and fresh basil on a plate.
2. Drizzle with balsamic glaze, olive oil, and season with salt and pepper.

9. Shrimp and Quinoa Salad

Serving: 1 salad
Nutritional Value
- Protein from shrimp
- Fiber and vitamins from quinoa and vegetables
- Healthy fats from avocado

Cooking Time: 20 minutes
Ingredients
- Grilled shrimp
- Cooked quinoa
- Mixed greens, cherry tomatoes, and cucumber
- Avocado slices
- Lemon vinaigrette dressing

Instructions
1. Combine grilled shrimp, cooked quinoa, mixed greens, cherry tomatoes, cucumber, and avocado slices in a bowl.
2. Drizzle with lemon vinaigrette dressing.

10. Vegetarian Lentil Soup

Serving: 1 bowl

Nutritional Value
- Protein and fiber from lentils
- Vitamins and minerals from vegetables
- Low in saturated fats

Cooking Time: 30 minutes

Ingredients
- Red lentils, rinsed
- Carrots, celery, and onion, diced
- Vegetable broth
- Garlic and cumin for seasoning
- Fresh parsley for garnish

Instructions

1. Sauté onions, carrots, and celery until softened.
2. Add lentils, vegetable broth, garlic, and cumin. Simmer until lentils are tender.
3. Garnish with fresh parsley before serving this hearty and nutritious soup.

Chapter 4: Colorful Dinner

1. Grilled Chicken and Vegetable Skewers

Serving: 1 plate

Nutritional Value
- Lean protein from chicken
- Fiber and vitamins from vegetables
- Healthy fats from olive oil

Cooking Time: 30 minutes

Ingredients
- Chicken breast, cut into cubes
- Bell peppers, cherry tomatoes, and red onion
- Garlic, herb & spicy and Olive oil for marinade
- Skewers for grilling

Instructions
1. Marinate chicken cubes and vegetables in olive oil, garlic, and herbs.
2. Thread onto skewers and grill until chicken is cooked.

3. Serve with a side of quinoa or brown rice.

2. Vegetarian Stuffed Bell Peppers

Serving: 1 pepper

Nutritional Value
- Quinoa and black beans protein
- Fiber and vitamins from vegetables
- Healthy fats from avocado

Cooking Time: 45 minutes

Ingredients
- Bell peppers, halved and cleaned
- Cooked quinoa
- Black beans, corn, diced tomatoes
- Avocado slices
- Mexican seasoning

Instructions

1. Mix quinoa, black beans, corn, diced tomatoes, and Mexican seasoning.
2. Stuff bell peppers with the mixture and bake until peppers are tender.
3. Top with avocado slices before serving.

3. Salmon and Asparagus Foil Packets

Serving: 1 packet

Nutritional Value

- Omega-3 fatty acids from salmon
- Fiber and vitamins from asparagus
- Healthy fats from olive oil

Cooking Time: 25 minutes

Ingredients:

- Salmon filet
- Asparagus spears
- Lemon slices, garlic, and dill for seasoning
- Olive oil

Instructions

1. Place salmon and asparagus on a foil sheet.
2. Season with lemon slices, garlic, dill, and drizzle with olive oil.
3. Seal the foil packet and bake until salmon is cooked through.

4. Eggplant and Chickpea Curry

Serving: 1 bowl

Nutritional Value
- Fiber and protein from chickpeas
- Antioxidants and vitamins from eggplant
- Healthy fats from coconut milk

Cooking Time: 40 minutes

Ingredients
- Eggplant, diced
- Chickpeas (canned, drained, and rinsed)
- Curry spices, coconut milk
- Brown rice or quinoa for serving

Instructions

1. Sauté eggplant until softened, add chickpeas, curry spices, and coconut milk.
2. Simmer until flavors meld, and serve over brown rice or quinoa.

5. Turkey and Vegetable Stir-Fry

Serving: 1 bowl

Nutritional Value
- Lean protein from turkey
- Fiber and vitamins from vegetables
- Healthy fats from sesame oil

Cooking Time: 20 minutes

Ingredients
- Ground turkey
- Broccoli florets, bell peppers, and snap peas
- Soy sauce, garlic, and ginger for seasoning
- Sesame oil

Instructions

1. Brown ground turkey in sesame oil, add vegetables, soy sauce, garlic, and ginger.
2. Stir-fry until turkey is cooked, and vegetables are tender.
3. Serve over brown rice or quinoa.

6. Cauliflower and Chickpea Curry

Serving: 1 bowl

Nutritional Value
- Fiber and protein from chickpeas
- Vitamins and antioxidants from cauliflower
- Healthy fats from coconut milk

Cooking Time: 30 minutes

Ingredients
- Cauliflower florets
- Chickpeas (canned, drained, and rinsed)
- Curry spices, coconut milk
- Basmati rice for serving

Instructions
1. Sauté cauliflower until lightly browned, add chickpeas, curry spices, and coconut milk.
2. Simmer until cauliflower is tender, and serve over basmati rice.

7. Shrimp and Zucchini Noodles

Serving: 1 plate
Nutritional Value
- Protein from shrimp
- Fiber and vitamins from zucchini noodles
- Healthy fats from olive oil

Cooking Time: 20 minutes
Ingredients
- Shrimp, peeled and deveined
- Zucchini, spiralized into noodles
- Garlic, lemon juice, and red pepper flakes for seasoning
- Olive oil

Instructions
1. Sauté shrimp in olive oil with garlic, red pepper flakes, and lemon juice.
2. Add zucchini noodles and cook until tender.
3. Serve this light and flavorful dish.

8. Chickpea and Spinach Stew

Serving: 1 bowl

Nutritional Value
- Fiber and protein from chickpeas
- Iron and vitamins from spinach
- Healthy fats from olive oil

Cooking Time: 35 minutes

Ingredients

- Chickpeas (canned, drained, and rinsed)
- Fresh spinach leaves
- Tomatoes, diced
- Garlic, onion, and cumin for seasoning
- Olive oil

Instructions

1. Sauté garlic and onion in olive oil, add chickpeas, tomatoes, and cumin.
2. Simmer until flavors meld, stir in fresh spinach until wilted.
3. Serve as a hearty and nutritious stew.

9. Teriyaki Tofu Stir-Fry

Serving: 1 bowl

Nutritional Value
- Plant-based protein from tofu
- Fiber and vitamins from vegetables
- Healthy fats from sesame oil

Cooking Time: 25 minutes

Ingredients
- Tofu, cubed
- Broccoli florets, bell peppers, and carrots
- Teriyaki sauce
- Sesame oil

Instructions

1. Sauté tofu in sesame oil until golden, add vegetables and teriyaki sauce.
2. Stir-fry until vegetables are tender, and tofu is coated.
3. Serve over brown rice or quinoa.

10. Mushroom and Lentil Stuffed Peppers

Serving: 1 pepper

Nutritional Value
- Protein and fiber from lentil
- Vitamins and minerals from mushrooms
- Healthy fats from olive oil

Cooking Time: 45 minutes

Ingredients
- Lentils, cooked
- Mushrooms, diced
- Bell peppers, halved and cleaned
- Onion, garlic, and Italian herbs for seasoning
- Olive oil

Instructions

1. Sauté mushrooms, onion, and garlic in olive oil, add cooked lentils and herbs.
2. Stuff bell peppers with the lentil and mushroom mixture.
3. Bake until peppers are tender, and serve with a side salad.

Chapter 4: Nutrient-rich Snacks

1. Greek Yogurt and Berry Parfait

Serving: 1 parfait

Nutritional Value
- Protein from Greek yogurt
- Antioxidants and fiber from berries
- Healthy fats from granola and nuts

Prep Time: 5 minutes

Ingredients
- 1/2 cup Greek yogurt
- Mixed berries (blueberries, strawberries)
- 2 tablespoons granola (low sugar)
- 1 tablespoon chopped nuts (almonds, walnuts)

Instructions
1. In a glass, layer Greek yogurt, mixed berries, granola, and chopped nuts.
2. Repeat the layers and enjoy a delicious and satisfying parfait.

2. Apple Slices with Almond Butter

Serving: 1 snack
Nutritional Value
- Fiber from apple slices
- Protein and healthy fats from almond butter

Prep Time: 5 minutes
Ingredients
- Apple, sliced
- 2 tablespoons almond butter

Instructions
1. Spread almond butter on apple slices.
2. Enjoy this quick and nutrient-rich snack for a balance of sweetness and crunch.

3. Vegetable Sticks with Hummus

Serving: 1 snack

Nutritional Value
- Fiber and vitamins from vegetables
- Protein and healthy fats from hummus

Prep Time: 10 minutes

Ingredients
- Carrot and cucumber sticks
- Cherry tomatoes
- Hummus for dipping

Instructions

1. Arrange vegetable sticks and cherry tomatoes on a plate.
2. Dip in hummus for a refreshing and nutritious snack.

4. Hard-Boiled Eggs with Avocado

Serving: 1 snack
Nutritional Value
 - Protein from eggs
 - Healthy fats from avocado

Prep Time: 10 minutes
Ingredients
- 2 hard-boiled eggs
- 1/2 avocado, sliced
- Salt, pepper, and a sprinkle of paprika for tasting

Instructions
1. Cut hard-boiled eggs in half.
2. Top each half with slices of avocado, and season with salt, pepper, and paprika.

5. Trail Mix

Serving: 1 handful
Nutritional Value
- Protein from nuts
- Fiber from dried fruits
- Healthy fats from seeds

Prep Time: 5 minutes
Ingredients
- Almonds, walnuts, and pistachios
- Dried cranberries or raisins
- Pumpkin seeds

Instructions
1. Mix almonds, walnuts, pistachios, dried cranberries or raisins, and pumpkin seeds.
2. Portion out a handful for a convenient and satisfying snack.

6. Cottage Cheese with Pineapple

Serving: 1 snack
Nutritional Value
- Protein from cottage cheese
- Vitamins and enzymes from pineapple

Prep Time: 5 minutes
Ingredients
- 1/2 cup low-fat cottage cheese
- Fresh pineapple chunks

Instructions
1. Combine cottage cheese with fresh pineapple chunks.

2. Enjoy this tropical-flavored snack for a dose of protein and sweetness.

7. Rice Cake with Almond Butter and Banana Slices

Serving: 1 snack
Nutritional Value
- Fiber from rice cake
- Protein and healthy fats from almond butter
- Potassium and vitamins from banana slices

Prep Time: 5 minutes
Ingredients
- Rice cake
- 1 tablespoon almond butter
- Banana slices

Instructions
1. Spread almond butter on a rice cake.
2. Top with banana slices for a crunchy and satisfying snack.

8. Yogurt-Dipped Strawberries

Serving: 1 snack
Nutritional Value
- Protein from yogurt
- Antioxidants and fiber from strawberries

Prep Time: 10 minutes
Ingredients
- Fresh strawberries
- Greek yogurt

Instructions
1. Dip strawberries in Greek yogurt.
2. Place on a tray and freeze for a refreshing and guilt-free treat.

9. Edamame Pods

Serving: 1 snack
Nutritional Value
- Protein and fiber from edamame
- Vitamins and minerals

Prep Time: 5 minutes
Ingredients
- Edamame pods (frozen, thawed)

Instructions
1. Steam or boil edamame pods until tender.
2. Sprinkle with a pinch of salt and enjoy this nutritious and fun-to-eat snack.

10. Dark Chocolate and Almond Clusters

Serving: 1 cluster
Nutritional Value
- Antioxidants from dark chocolate
- Protein and healthy fats from almonds

Prep Time: 15 minutes
Ingredients
- Dark chocolate squares
- Almonds

Instructions
1. Melt dark chocolate and mix with almonds.
2. Spoon clusters onto parchment paper and let them set in the refrigerator.
3. Savor these indulgent yet health-conscious chocolate-almond clusters.

Chapter 6: Bonus 1: 7-day meal plan

Day 1

Breakfast: Quinoa Breakfast Bowl with Berries and Almonds
Lunch: Grilled Chicken and Vegetable Salad with Olive Oil Dressing
Snack: Greek Yogurt and Berry Parfait
Dinner: Salmon and Asparagus Foil Packets with Quinoa

Day 2

Breakfast: Chia Seed Pudding with Fresh Berries
Lunch: Chickpea and Spinach Stew with Brown Rice
Snack: Vegetable Sticks with Hummus
Dinner: Basmati rice and Chickpeas with Eggplant

Day 3

Breakfast: Peanut Butter Banana Overnight Oats
Lunch: Turkey and Quinoa Stuffed Bell Peppers
Snack: Apple Slices with Almond Butter
Dinner: Teriyaki Tofu Stir-Fry with Brown Rice

Day 4

Breakfast: Greek Yogurt Parfait with Mixed Berries and Chia Seeds
Lunch: Shrimp and Quinoa Salad with Avocado
Snack: Trail Mix (Nuts, Seeds, Dried Fruits)
Dinner: Vegetarian Lentil Soup with a Side Salad

Day 5

Breakfast: Avocado and Egg Toast on Whole Grain Bread

Lunch: Caprese Salad with Balsamic Glaze

Snack: Cottage Cheese with Pineapple Chunks

Dinner: Mushroom and Lentil Stuffed Peppers

Day 6

Breakfast: Berry and Almond Smoothie Bowl

Lunch: Sweet Potato and Chickpea Buddha Bowl

Snack: Rice Cake with Almond Butter and Banana Slices

Dinner: Chicken and Vegetable Stir-Fry with Quinoa

Day 7

Breakfast: Vegetable Omelet with Spinach and Feta Cheese
Lunch: Mediterranean Hummus Plate with Whole Wheat Pita
Snack: Dark Chocolate and Almond Clusters
Dinner: Grilled Salmon Salad with Quinoa

Chapter 7: Bonus 2: Insulin resistance Juicing and Smoothie Recipes for seniors

1. Green Detox Juice

Ingredients: Spinach, cucumber, celery, green apple, lemon.

Instructions: Run all ingredients through a juicer and enjoy this refreshing detoxifying drink.

2. Beetroot Blast

Ingredients: Beetroot, carrot, ginger, apple.

Instructions: Juice the ingredients together for a vibrant and antioxidant-rich beverage.

3. Citrus Burst Juice

Ingredients: Oranges, grapefruits, lemon.

Instructions: Extract juice from citrus fruits for a zesty and vitamin C-packed drink.

4. Carrot-Orange Elixir

Ingredients: Carrots, oranges.

Instructions: Combine carrots and oranges for a sweet and vitamin A-rich elixir.

5. Cucumber Mint Cooler

Ingredients: Cucumber, mint, lime.

Instructions: Juicer all ingredients and experience a hydrating and refreshing drink.

6. Berry Bliss Smoothie

Ingredients: Mixed berries (strawberries, blueberries, raspberries), Greek yogurt, almond milk.

Instructions: Blend together for a delicious and antioxidant-filled smoothie.

7. Pineapple Paradise

Ingredients: Pineapple, banana, coconut water.

Instructions: Blend for a tropical and hydrating smoothie.

8. Green Power Smoothie

Ingredients: Kale, banana, green apple, chia seeds, almond milk.

Instructions: Blend for a nutrient-dense and fiber-rich green smoothie.

9. Avocado Delight

Ingredients: Avocado, spinach, mango, lime, water.

Instructions: Create a creamy and satisfying smoothie with this combination.

10. Mango Tango Smoothie

Ingredients: Mango, pineapple, Greek yogurt, coconut milk.

Instructions: Blend for a tropical and protein-packed smoothie.

11. Berries and Oats Smoothie

Ingredients: Mixed berries, rolled oats, almond milk, honey.

Instructions: Blend for a filling and fiber-rich smoothie.

12. Chia-Berry Protein Smoothie

Ingredients: Mixed berries, chia seeds, protein powder, almond milk.

Instructions: Blend for a protein-packed smoothie with added omega-3 from chia seeds.

13. Spinach and Banana Smoothie

Ingredients: Spinach, banana, almond milk, cinnamon.

Instructions: Create a simple and nutritious green smoothie with this combination.

14. Kiwi-Citrus Crush

Ingredients: Kiwi, orange, banana, Greek yogurt.

Instructions: Blend for a vitamin C boost and a creamy texture from yogurt.

15. Strawberry Almond Bliss

Ingredients: Strawberries, almond butter, almond milk.

Instructions: Blend for a nutty and berry-infused smoothie.

16. Turmeric Golden Smoothie

Ingredients: Pineapple, banana, turmeric, ginger, coconut water.

Instructions: Combine for an anti-inflammatory and tropical-flavored smoothie.

17. Peachy Green Smoothie

Ingredients: Peaches, spinach, Greek yogurt, water.

Instructions: Blend for a peachy and nutrient-packed green smoothie.

18. Blueberry Lavender Refresher

Ingredients: Blueberries, lavender, banana, almond milk.

Instructions: Create a unique and aromatic smoothie with blueberries and lavender.

19. Apple Pie Smoothie

Ingredients: Apple, cinnamon, oats, almond milk.

Instructions: Blend for a tasty smoothie reminiscent of apple pie.

20. Pomegranate Berry Blast

Ingredients: Pomegranate seeds, mixed berries, Greek yogurt, water.

Instructions: Blend for a vibrant and antioxidant-rich smoothie.

Conclusion

In the symphony of flavors and nutrition, these recipes strive to compose a harmonious balance for those navigating the path of insulin resistance. As you embark on this culinary journey, may these dishes become not just meals but companions in your pursuit of health and vitality. Remember, every bite is a choice, and every choice is a step toward nourishing your body, mind, and spirit. May the joy of wholesome eating be your constant guide, and may each delicious creation bring you closer to a life filled with wellness and happiness. Bon appétit, and here's to a future filled with vibrant health and culinary delight!

Printed in Great Britain
by Amazon